Traditional Vietnamese Medicine

MICHELLE TRAM

CONTENTS

DISCLAIMER

This book does not substitute for any professional medical advice or treatment. The information compiled in this book is solely intended to give insight into Traditional Vietnamese Medicine, as such practices may not be discussed as widely in public or healthcare settings. References have been cited at the end of the book to properly accredit said information.

INTRODUCTION: A BRIEF HISTORY OF TRADITIONAL VIETNAMESE MEDICINE

Traditional Vietnamese Medicine (Y học cổ truyền Việt Nam) originated in the rice valleys spanning the Red River, home to humble leaf-hatted farmers and the center of continuous Chinese conquest. Due to Chinese occupation by the Han, Sui, Tang, and Ming dynasties, Vietnamese medicine (Thuốc Nam) has been influenced by Chinese practices (Thuốc Bắc). The two may be dissimilar in that Vietnamese medicine focuses on raw, fresh herbs in contrast to more complex Chinese decoctions;[1] however, the underlying beliefs in traditional Vietnamese medicine is deeply interwoven with the heart of Chinese culture.

Both eastern medical practices harness an understanding of Qi, a universal energy stored in each person's body. Qi is obtained through biological inheritance and consumption of food. Eastern tradition emphasizes its significance for body movement, physical growth and development, and body defense mechanisms against pathological processes. However, since Qi is universal, it can easily become lost to an individual's surroundings. This belief highlights the necessity of spiritual exercises to regain the lost Qi from the universe and restore and maintain one's wellness.

In addition to the Qi, Vietnamese and Chinese medical practices are founded upon beliefs of yin and yang: two opposite but complementary forces within the body. To maintain healthy equilibrium, one must ensure a balance between the yin (representative of the cold, interior, deficiency) and yang (representative of the hot, exterior, excess). Distinct herbs and different foods—whether sour, bitter, sweet, spicy, or salty—can be consumed to treat each distinct yin or yang illness, help to regulate the flow of Qi in the body, and influence the balance of the body's five elements: wood, fire, earth, metal, and water. All elements are dependent upon each other to create balance, as deficiency in one element can lead to deficiency or excess of another element.[2]

Then, in 1887, under Napoleon III, France conquered Vietnam. The French introduced Western medicine (Thuốc Tây) to the subjugated Vietnamese.

The Vietnamese, in fervor for political independence, sought to distinguish their medical practices from an alien Western culture. In anti-colonial sentiment, the Vietnamese began to regard their medicine as Thuốc Ta, or "Our Medicine." In 1955, President Hồ Chí Minh hoped to achieve Vietnamese nationalism under his Democratic Republic of Vietnam, urging his people to "build [their] own medicine," by combining Western and Eastern medicine to enhance Traditional Vietnamese Medicine (TVM).[3]

Today, Traditional Vietnamese Medicine has diffused into the American lifestyle, absorbed by those perhaps disillusioned with modern medical practices and thus seeking an alternative remedy to the stresses of urbanization and modernity. As TVM has influenced Western medicine, so too has Western technology improved traditional herbal remedies. Despite the seemingly universal dominance of new medical advancements, many patients retain beliefs in Qi, yin and yang, and the five elements and continue to receive treatment under TVM.

However, due to the potential stigma associated with TVM and fear of disapproval from physicians, many Vietnamese-Americans are reluctant to share their experiences. This book has been written to educate about various types of TVM to spread more awareness about the subject into the general population. By increasing knowledge about TVM, communication and a mutual understanding between patients and their healthcare practitioners can definitely be enhanced.

WIND SNATCHING *(DẬT GIÓ)*

One traditional Vietnamese belief exists in the "toxic wind," or *Gió Độc,* that disrupts one's natural balance of the yin and yang. Thus, many interpret their illnesses, such as a cold or flu, to be disorders caused by excess wind, or "catching the wind" *(trúng gió).* In efforts to expel this wind from the body, the Vietnamese repeatedly use their fingers to pinch the skin and snap away, releasing the skin back to its original shape. Wind snatching is commonly performed in between the eyebrows to relieve headache or on the neck to aid neck pain or nausea.[4]

There exists a small number of studies that provide evidence for the efficacy of this procedure in reducing pain. On the other hand, wind snatching can irritate the skin, leading to skin infections and excessive skin bruising.

WIND SCRAPING *(CẠO GIÓ)*

Similar to the practice of wind snatching, wind scraping, which mirrors the Chinese *gua sha*, is believed to expunge the poisonous wind in one's body.[5] Often performed by patients themselves or by family members in a domestic setting, wind scraping utilizes coins or other dull instruments to make scraping motions directly on the skin. For back or stomach pain, the coin is stroked in a downward diagonal motion on one's back. For chest pain, the scraping is done in a diagonal, wheel-spoke pattern parallel to the ribs. It is believed that the intensity of the red color from scraping is positively correlated with the severity of the toxic wind. In other words, the deepest red streaks would denote the site of the most constricted muscles.[4] These red marks are created by the rupturing of tiny blood vessels at the surface of the skin where the coin is dragged. These bruise-like injuries, which can take approximately three to seven days to heal, are often mistaken for signs of physical abuse.[6] This plausible misperception can discourage many Vietnamese patients from sharing their traditional practices with their healthcare providers.

Over the years, wind scraping has garnered medical attention from numerous scientific experiments that hope to provide support for or against the effectiveness of the procedure. According to the *South China Morning Post* (SCMP), two Harvard studies have been done: the first concludes that wind scraping can stimulate anti-inflammatory responses and specifically treat liver inflammation in patients with chronic active hepatitis B, and the second demonstrates how wind scraping can enhance the body's immune system and thus augment the effectiveness of antibiotics. The same SCMP article also notes a 2012 study published in the *American Journal of Chinese Medicine* that tested patients with chronic neck pain. This study found that patients treated with wind scraping experienced less pain than did the control group.[6] The results of this research corroborates a 2011 German study, which discovered that neck pain decreased significantly more in patients treated with wind scraping than those treated with a neck heating pad.[7] One study attributes this reduction of pain and myalgia to an increase in microcirculation from coining.[8] More recently, a 2017 study in the *Menopause Journal* saw a positive relationship between wind scraping and the reduction of perimenopausal symptoms in women, including insomnia, headache, and sweating.[9] However, whether wind scraping yields long-term results remains unclear.

On the other hand, wind scraping has detrimental effects, such as raising the risk of infection. An instrument that is not properly sterilized can aid the contamination of pathogens through blood cells and fluids transmitted from one patient to another.[10]

CUPPING *(GIÁC HƠI)*

Cupping involves the placement of circular suction cups of glass or bamboo onto the patient's back, chest, or joints, in order to "suck out" the poisonous wind, which is believed to cause both acute and chronic pain. To create a suction inside of each cup, a lighted alcohol cotton ball is quickly waved in the cup to remove oxygen. Before the cups are placed onto the patient, the skin is lubricated with oils, allowing the therapist to easily move the cups along the affected area during the procedure.[4] Cups are generally placed along the five meridian lines, or the channels through which one's energy flows. The cups sit for five to ten minutes and are then snapped off, leaving behind red marks that can last up to three weeks. It is believed that the greater the discoloration, the more severe the level of toxins. Wet cupping differs from dry cupping in that the therapist makes small cuts on the skin before applying the cup onto the skin; this additional step allows the suction to draw out small amounts of blood.[11]

Many Olympic athletes, including swimmer Michael Phelps and gymnast Alexander Naddour, have turned to this traditional practice in the belief that cupping helps to relieve soreness after training sessions.[12] As cupping presumably draws up stagnant blood and sticky proteins that accumulate from muscular injuries, patients can experience stimulated circulation, ushering a faster recovery.[13] Indeed, a number of studies support the effectiveness of cupping in reducing pain from acne, cervical spondylosis, carpal tunnel syndrome, and facial paralysis, among many others.[12] Cupping can induce feelings of relaxation, leading to a higher level of endogenous opioids in the brain.[14] The increased production of these enkephalins and endorphins blocks pain signals in the spinal cord and brainstem, respectively, thereby allowing a patient to tolerate greater levels of pain.[15] A different study in Saudi Arabia in 2015 found that wet cupping can help lower the systolic blood pressure of patients with hypertension and thus minimize the risk for atherosclerosis.[16] However, other researchers note the problems in scientific methodologies such as biases and limited information provided from subjects involved in the studies. Critics to these studies also point to the placebo effect, attributing patients' reduction of pain to their psychological belief in the treatment, rather than the effectiveness of the treatment itself. Thus, they determine that these previous studies alone are insufficient to formulate a definite conclusion regarding the health benefits of cupping.

One should also be aware of the complications associated with cupping. Due to the usage of fire, the risk for skin burns is high. In addition, if the cupping procedure is not properly supervised or performed, the vacuum can cause painful blisters at the site.[12] Some patients experience skin pigmentation and nausea, along with bruises from broken capillaries. Furthermore, infection, thrombocytopenia (low levels of blood platelets), and transmission of diseases, such as hepatitis, can occur with wet cupping.[17]

BLOODLETTING *(CẮT LỂ)*

Bloodletting is an ancient medical practice shared by ancient Egyptian, European, and Asian cultures. In TVM, bloodletting focuses specifically on removing the poisonous wind in a patient's blood. Often using a shard of glass or small razor blade, the patient pinches and performs small cuts on the skin, removing blood by squeezing the site of incision.[4] Bloodletting is often incorporated in other traditional medical procedures, such as in cupping.

In western medicine, doctors prescribe phlebotomy therapy to remove excess blood to treat rare cases of polycythemia, a blood condition involving an abnormally high number of red blood cells that can "thicken" a patient's blood and thus increase the risk of heart attack and stroke. In addition, phlebotomy therapy is used to treat hemochromatosis.[18] Hemochromatosis is a disorder where excess iron can cause liver disease and heart complications. Furthermore, a small 2012 *BioMed Central Medicine* study found that blood pressure and cholesterol levels improved in subjects who donated up to a pint of blood, in comparison to those who did not.[19]

Nevertheless, bloodletting can be dangerous if it depletes too much of the body's iron supply, which is necessary in the formation of hemoglobin, a protein in red blood cells that carries oxygen throughout the body. A sudden loss of large amounts of blood can invoke hypotensive shock, stroke, major organ failure, or cardiac arrest. In addition to leaving scars, bloodletting can lead to infections if the instruments or wounds are contaminated or unclean.[18] Infections from tetanus bacteria are common due to their natural ubiquity in the environment. Tetanus attacks the body's central nervous system and can cause fever, severe lockjaw, painful muscle spasm, and death.

ACUPUNCTURE *(CHÂM CỨU)*

Early acupuncture used lances to cut veins along meridian lines in order to restore the flow of Qi and was later developed to use needles. By inserting needles into a patient's subcutaneous tissue at specific acupuncture points, traditional acupuncturists believe they can promote a balance between the patient's yin and yang forces, thereby stimulating a healthy flow of Qi. Patients turn to acupuncture for many health conditions, but most commonly for neck pain, arthritis, and headaches.[20]

Western scientists believe that acupuncture works to increase the production of endorphins in the body by stimulating specific nerves as the needles are applied. These endorphins trigger feelings of happiness, increasing a patient's pain threshold. In addition to increasing the production of endorphins, acupuncture has been found to decrease the number of pro-inflammatory cytokines in the body. In a 2003 study, researchers applied acupuncture to a group of patients with chronic headache; results revealed that proinflammatory interleukin(IL)-1beta, IL-6, and tumor necrosis factor-alpha levels decreased after treatment.[21] By reducing inflammation, acupuncture mitigates pain. Other scientists attribute the effectiveness of acupuncture to its ability to stimulate the secretion of nerve growth factor, thereby promoting the regeneration of nerve cells.[22]

In addition to relieving pain, acupuncture has been shown to restore hormonal balance by regulating ovulation, thereby increasing the chances of a successful pregnancy.[23] Furthermore, a 2017 study found that acupuncture can help alleviate symptoms of posttraumatic stress disorder, such as depression.[24] However, many researchers acknowledge the methodology limitations of these studies, suggesting the need for more and better designed studies.

The benefits of acupuncture tend to be short-term, while the risks, although low, merit consideration. Similar to bloodletting and any medical procedure that inserts instruments into a patient's body, infection is plausible if the equipment has not been properly sterilized. Negligent acupuncture can lead to hepatitis, tuberculosis, mycobacterium, and methicillin-resistant Staphylococcus aureus (MRSA) infection. In addition, deep needling can puncture blood vessels and lead to hematoma, which involves the abnormal collection of clotting blood in the injured tissue.[25] Thus, caution should be taken to mitigate any risks in which patients may endure organ, vascular, or nerve injury, especially near the thoracic and abdominal areas. Lastly, rare cases occur in which silver dislodges from the needle into the patient's body, leading to argyria, or skin discoloration due to exposure to insoluble silver.[25]

ACUPRESSURE *(BẤM HUYỆT)*

Similar to acupuncture, acupressure centers on the belief of Qi, seeking to rechannel this energy along the meridians to restore the body to its natural state of health. Acupressurists apply pressure onto the affected areas with their finger tips. Other therapists may use other objects, such as small electric vibrators, to stimulate the acupressure points.[4] To relieve symptoms of headache, low energy, and eye fatigue, patients would apply acupressure to the back of the neck, near their mastoid (ear) bone, and to their shoulder muscles. To relieve stress, patients massage the area between the thumb and index finger on the hand, as well as the region between the big toe and the second toe on the foot. Patients can also apply pressure to the inner forearm and beneath the kneecap to relieve nausea and stomachache, while pressing above the ankle bone to treat menstrual cramps and urological problems.[26]

Many studies provide support for the effectiveness of acupressure in relieving pain. One 2004 study tested two groups of patients with lower back pain: one group was treated with four weeks of acupressure and was compared with a control group who only underwent physical therapy. Follow-up assessments concluded that the patients who were treated with acupressure felt less pain.[27] A 2008 study tested acupressure at the "extra 1" point, or the Yin Tang point between the eyebrows. Here, acupressure induces sedation, as it decreases bispectral index (BIS) values, signifying high levels of hypnosis.[28] By contributing to a patient's hypnotic state, acupressure consequently stimulates the parasympathetic nervous system, which is responsible for relaxing the body.[29, 30]

Auricular point acupressure (APA), which concentrates on points on the inner and outer ear lobe, has been shown to reduce the levels of proinflammatory cytokines IL-1beta, IL-2, and IL-6, thereby lessening pain. In fact, the recent 2014 study reported a 56% reduction in pain in the APA group, in comparison to a 9% reduction in pain in the control group, where sham APA was performed.[31]

However, since the primary meridian points can be located at sensitive private areas, such as near the pelvic bone or across the chest, a patient may feel uncomfortable during the acupressure procedure.

MOXIBUSTION *(MOXIB PHỔNG)*

Moxibustion, a form of heat therapy originating during the pre-Qin dynasty in China, involves the burning of rolled moxa leaves, or dried mugwort, and can be divided into direct and indirect moxibustion. Direct moxibustion entails the direct placement of burning moxa onto the patient's skin at acupuncture points. This type of moxibustion can be further differentiated between scarring and non-scarring. The former yields visual cues such as blistering and scarring before removal, whereas the latter ends the procedure before scarring can occur. On the other hand, in indirect moxibustion, the burning material is held close to, yet not touching, the patient's skin.[32] Moxa, a pungent herb easily and abundantly grown throughout Asia, is believed to warm the meridians, thereby promoting circulation and relieving pain from arthritis or the cold; this distinctive herbal quality distinguishes moxibustion from various other heating devices, such as heating pads.[33] In warming Yang, promoting Qi, and removing wind, traditional medicine practitioners see moxibustion as a successful treatment to diseases or illnesses that could not be fully treated by acupuncture alone. Unlike acupuncture, moxibustion is often performed at home by patients themselves as an easy supplement to clinical treatment.[34] Using modern technology, moxibustion has evolved in the clinical sphere to include microwave, laser, and electrothermal moxibustion.

Burning moxa produces shortened infrared wavelengths that trigger notable photochemical changes. These shortened wavelengths are able to deeply penetrate tissues, in comparison to normal infrared radiation. When mitochondria absorbs red light, cellular metabolism is enhanced, thereby increasing protein synthesis, which is necessary for the functioning of a cell and healing of tissue. In addition, red light promotes phagocytosis, a process in which cells of the immune system engulf other cells to protect the body against infectious or invading agents. The light energy is also absorbed by water in cells where it transforms into kinetic energy and increases the water temperature. As a result, blood is able to travel more quickly, enhancing blood circulation.[35] One study even concluded that moxibustion was as successful as the sedative estazolam in combating insomnia.[36] Another experiment tested indirect moxibustion on patients with chronic kidney disease and found that renal vascular resistance, or the impediment of blood flow in kidney blood vessels, decreased after treatment.[37] These recorded health benefits can be attributed to the red and near infrared radiation from moxibustion.

The smoke from the burning mugwort produces a lingering smell resembling the odor of marijuana.[33] Patients with sensitive smell, for example cancer patients undergoing chemotherapy, can experience symptoms of nausea and vomiting, as well as other gastrointestinal issues. More concerning are the ramifications of inhaling excessive amounts of the smoke. Patients can experience difficulty breathing, tightness in the chest, and allergies when undergoing moxibustion in a poorly ventilated room. In addition, moxa smoke is found to contain polycyclic aromatic carcinogens and an increased amount of air pollutants, such as nitrogen oxides and particulates. In direct moxibustion, the most common complication is burns, which induce painful blisters and infections, as well as permanent scarring.[38] However, these problems are mostly associated with the ill performance of moxibustion, due to lack of practitioner skill or patient-practitioner miscommunication.

TIGER BALM *(DẦU CÙ LÀ)*

Tiger balm is a topical ointment applied to various parts of the body to treat body discomfort, including headaches, back and joint pain, burns, and stomachaches. Patients apply this medication by massaging the balm into the skin until the substance is absorbed. Generally, a cooling sensation follows, relieving the patient of any sensation of pain. Many Vietnamese-Americans can recall the widespread uses of this essential product in their household, inciting memories of their grandparents who had introduced the balm generations earlier. The main active ingredients in tiger balm include methyl salicylate, which helps numb the skin; menthol, which increases blood circulation through dilating blood vessels; and camphor, which similarly stimulates blood flow to reduce swelling and inflammation.[39]

Tiger balm's widespread success can be attributed to the efficacy of its ingredients. In 2014, a group of scientists studied the effects of camphor on blood flow. The scientists deduced a positive correlation between camphor and the production of nitric oxide (NO) to explain the sustained increase of skin and muscle blood flow after applications of increased concentrations of camphor.[40] Specifically, NO is responsible for vasodilation, a process in which blood vessels relax and dilate, allowing for easy movement of blood through these channels.[41] In addition, menthol has been found to raise subjects' cough thresholds when tested against a control placebo. These subjects were less sensitive to inhaled capsaicin.[42] Lastly, a study tested both men and women with muscle pain by treating the group with skin patches composed of methyl salicylate and menthol. Results showed that after an 8-hour application of these patches, patients experienced significantly less pain compared with those treated with placebo.[43]

Despite these benefits, tiger balm usage must be monitored closely, as excessive application of any ingredient can cause intolerable skin irritation. In 2007, high school athlete Arielle Newman accidentally overdosed on methyl salicylate due to excessive use of a variety of muscle creams and died as a result. When topically applied to over forty percent of the body or used by an individual with specific skin conditions or in conjunction with other products, methyl salicylate can prove detrimental.[44] However, these cases are rare and tiger balm continues to be a widespread household medicine.

HOT WATER FOOT BATH *(NGẮM CHẤN NƯỚC NÓNG)*

Inspired by the ancient Chinese, those practicing Traditional Vietnamese Medicine often prepare hot water foot baths. The foot is believed to be the site of six meridians, specifically the gall bladder, kidney, spleen, liver, and stomach. Thus, by soaking one's feet in hot water, the heat is believed to activate blood and energy channels throughout the body. Sweating is often a good sign that one's energy channels are being cleared; however, when the body begins to sweat, it is advised to remove the feet from the bath. Too much sweating is interpreted to mean that the body is using up too much energy.[45]

Different herbs are often used in foot baths, including ginger, for their medicinal qualities. For example, ginger is believed to be able to restore yang by warming the body, thereby reducing body pains, as well as symptoms from the common cold.[46] In addition, epsom salt (which differs from table salt due to its pure composition of magnesium and sulfate) can be dissolved into the water. During foot baths, the magnesium in the epsom salt can be absorbed by the skin,[47, 48] which can help decrease inflammation by acting as a calcium channel blocker (calcium is a pro-inflammatory mineral).[49] However, the National Institutes of Health raises a credible concern against the magnesium in epsom salts: high amounts of magnesium can cause an increase in insulin release, which can be dangerous for those with diabetes.[50] In addition, high levels of magnesium can cause a variety of side effects, such as low blood pressure and muscle weakness.[51]

Similar to the effects of other forms of heat therapy, the hot water from the foot bath stimulates blood flow to areas of stiffness.[50] Edema, which involves swelling caused by excess fluids trapped in the tissue, can be treated by the hot water, which can help decrease pain and inflammation.[52]

Despite the claims of proponents, many critics argue against the ability of epsom salts in drawing out toxins from the body. Although some may attribute the removal of toxins through the process of osmosis (believing that toxins can leave the body through the skin), critics are quick to address the inaccuracy of this statement: only the water moves through the skin in osmosis.[53] In addition, claims regarding the absorption of magnesium transdermally still warrants more research.

EUCALYPTUS OIL *(KHUYNH DIỆP)*

A native plant to Australia, the eucalyptus tree produces an oil commonly used in TVM topical ointments. The main species of eucalyptus grown for its medicinal qualities is *Eucalyptus globulus*, or commonly known as Blue Gum. Popular for its sharp smell of mint and honey, many people continue to use eucalyptus oil to treat symptoms of colds and coughs, as well as for various muscle pains.

One study points towards the antibacterial effects of eucalyptus when tested on pathogenic bacteria in the respiratory tract.[54] Specifically, eucalyptus oil was tested on rats, where it succeeded in stimulating an immune system response to pathogens in vivo. The study also tested eucalyptus oil on human monocyte derived macrophages (MDMs) in vitro, finding that their phagocytic responses were bolstered and the amount of released pro-inflammatory cytokines lessened.[55] In addition, eucalyptus oil has been studied as a natural antibiotic to prevent infectious diseases caused by the bacteria *E. coli* and *S. aureus*.[56] *E. coli* is associated with urinary tract infections and *S. aureus* is most responsible for post-operative wound infections. Eucalyptus oil has also demonstrated its efficacy in reducing pain and inflammation when applied to patients recovering from knee replacement surgery.[57]

Eucalyptus oil should be applied carefully, avoiding sensitive areas such as around the eyes, in order to prevent irritation. This essential oil must be diluted before application. In addition, as eucalyptus is highly allergenic as well as toxic, patients must take precaution before applying ointments with eucalyptus extract.[58] As eucalyptus oil can cause seizures if accidentally swallowed,[59] it is important to monitor usage in young children or the uninformed.

BOILING HERBS *(XÔNG HƠI)*

Often, Vietnamese patients boil various types
of herbs for their distinct medicinal properties. For
example, they may boil lemongrass *(cộng sả)* to make
tea purported to treat anxiety and stress or to prevent
infections. Although more studies are needed to
justify the calming effects of lemongrass, research has
shown that lemongrass can fight against
microorganisms, suggesting it to be a plausible
antifungal treatment.[60] In addition, in a study testing
the consumption of lemongrass tea on human
subjects, scientists conclude that this herb plays a role
in increasing hemoglobin concentration and the
amount of red blood cells in the body. These results
point to a potential solution to treat anemia.[61]
However, healthcare professionals warn against
consuming lemongrass if one is currently undergoing
chemotherapy, as the herb can inhibit the

effectiveness of some medication. In addition, due to the possibility of birth defects (as seen in studies testing citral and myrcene, which are both components of lemongrass, in rats), pregnant women should be cautioned against consuming this herb.[60]

Another herb commonly boiled is Vietnamese coriander (*rau răm*). Different extracts of this herb, specifically methanol, n-hexane, and dichloromethane, have been tested against bacteria with antifungal and antibiotic controls. Although results showed that these extracts were inactive against fungi, scientists concluded that Vietnamese coriander extracts exhibit strong antibacterial properties.[62]

Ginger (*gừng*) is another herb boiled into tea and drank for its medicinal properties in reducing pain, inflammation, and nausea. A study performed by the University of Georgia found that the consistent consumption of ginger over the period of eleven days helped to reduce muscle pain by 25% in participants.[63] However, some minor side effects from consuming ginger water include gas and abdominal pain.[64]

REFERENCES

1. Roth, Sam. "The Ins and Outs of Traditional Vietnamese Medicine." *Culture Trip*, The Culture Trip, 5 Apr. 2018, theculturetrip.com/asia/vietnam/articles/the-ins-and-outs-of-traditional-vietnamese-medicine/.

2. Thai, Hue Chan. "Traditional Vietnamese Medicine: Historical Perspective and Current Usage." *EthnoMed*, 1 Aug. 2003, ethnomed.org/clinical/traditional-medicine/traditional-vietnamese-medicine-historical-perspective-and-current-usage.

3. Monnais, Laurence, et al. "Southern Medicine for Southern People." Introduction. *Southern Medicine for Southern People: Vietnamese Medicine*

in the Making, Cambridge Scholars, 2012, pp. 1-15. *Cambridge Scholars*, www.cambridgescholars.com/download/sample/60495.

4. Nguyen, Long T et al. "The Use of Traditional Vietnamese Medicine Among Vietnamese Immigrants Attending an Urban Community Health Center in the United States." *Journal of alternative and complementary medicine (New York, N.Y.)* vol. 22,2 (2016): 145-53. doi:10.1089/acm.2014.0209.

5. Pich, Lan. *Cao Gio (Coin Rubbing or Coining)*. Health Psychology, 14 Oct. 2006. *Health Psychology*, healthpsych.psy.vanderbilt.edu/CAOGIO.htm.

6. Snouffer, Elizabeth. "Traditional Chinese Medicine's Scraping Treatment Put to the Test." *South China Morning Post*, South China Morning Post, 9 Oct. 2017, 12:00 AM, www.scmp.com/lifestyle/health/article/1056423/traditional-chinese-medicines-scraping-treatment-put-test.

7. Braun, Maximilian, et al. "Effectiveness of Traditional Chinese 'Gua Sha' Therapy in

Patients with Chronic Neck Pain: A Randomized Controlled Trial." *Pain Medicine*, vol. 12, no. 3, Mar. 2011, doi:10.1111/j.1526-4637.2011.01053.x. Abstract.

8. Nielsen, Arya, et al. "The Effect of Gua Sha Treatment on the Microcirculation of Surface Tissue: A Pilot Study in Healthy Subjects." *The Journal of Science and Healing*, vol. 3, no. 5, Sept. 2007, doi:10.1016/j.explore.2007.06.001. Abstract.

9. Fang, Meng, et al. "Effect of Gua Sha Therapy on Perimenopausal Syndrome: A Randomized Controlled Trial." *Menopause*, vol. 24, no. 3, Mar. 2017, doi:10.1097/GME.0000000000000752. Abstract.

10. Sissons, Claire. "Gua Sha: Uses, Benefits, and Side Effects." Edited by Debra Rose Wilson, *Medical News Today*, MediLexicon International, 23 Dec. 2017, www.medicalnewstoday.com/articles/320397.php.

11. Vitale, Susan Ann, and Thaleshravi Prashad. "Cultural Awareness: Coining and Cupping." *International Archives of Nursing and Health Care*,

vol. 3, no. 3, 2017, doi:10.23937/2469-5823/1510080.

12. Wang, Jeanette. "Five Things You Should Know about Cupping, Chinese Medicine Therapy on View in Rio." *South China Morning Post*, South China Morning Post, 13 Aug. 2016, www.scmp.com/lifestyle/health-beauty/article/2002783/five-things-you-should-know-about-cupping-chinese-medicine.

13. "A Word on Cupping Marks." *Cupping Therapy Detoxification*, International Cupping Therapy Association, 2005, www.cuppingtherapy.org/pages/discolorations.htm.

14. Al-Bedah, Abdullah M N et al. "The medical perspective of cupping therapy: Effects and mechanisms of action." *Journal of traditional and complementary medicine* vol. 9,2 90-97. 30 Apr. 2018, doi:10.1016/j.jtcme.2018.03.003.

15. "Endorphin and Enkephalin." *Encyclopedia*, www.encyclopedia.com/medicine/ medical-journals/endorphin-and-enkephalin.

16. Aleyeidi, Nouran A., et al. "Effects of Wet-Cupping on Blood Pressure in Hypertensive

Patients: A Randomized Controlled Trial." *Journal of Integrative Medicine*, vol. 13, no. 6, Nov. 2015, doi:10.1016/S2095-4964(15)60197-2.

17. Wong, Cathy. "Cupping Therapy Overview, Benefits, and Side Effects." *Verywell Health*, Dotdash, 2 July 2019, www.verywellhealth.com/cupping-for-pain-88933.

18. Engelhaupt, Erika. "Bloodletting Is Still Happening, Despite Centuries of Harm." *National Geographic*, National Geographic, 27 Oct. 2015, www.nationalgeographic.com/science/pheno mena/2015/10/27/bloodletting-is-still-happening-despite-centuries-of-harm/.

19. Houschyar, Khosrow S., et al. "Effects of Phlebotomy-Induced Reduction of Body Iron Stores on Metabolic Syndrome: Results from a Randomized Clinical Trial." *BMC Medicine*, vol. 10, no. 54, 30 May 2012, doi:10.1186/1741-7015-10-54.

20. Cosio, David, and Erica H. Lin. "Traditional Chinese Medicine & Acupuncture." *Practical Pain Management*, vol. 15, no. 7, 16 May 2016, www.practicalpainmanagement.com/treatmen

ts/complementary/acupuncture/traditional-chinese-medicine-acupuncture.

21. Jeong, Hyun-Ja, et al. "The Effect of Acupuncture on Proinflammatory Cytokine Production in Patients with Chronic Headache: A Preliminary Report." *The American Journal of Chinese Medicine*, vol. 31, no. 6, 2003, doi:10.1142/S0192415X03001661.

22. Palermo, Elizabeth. "What Is Acupuncture?" *Live Science*, Purch, 21 June 2017, www.livescience.com/29494-acupuncture.html.

23. "Acupuncture For Fertility - Safely Increase Chance of Conception." *Pacific College of Oriental Medicine*, Pacific College of Oriental Medicine, 24 May 2019, www.pacificcollege.edu/news/blog/2015/04/17/how-does-acupuncture-fertility-work-increase-chance-conception-without-side-effects.

24. Grant, Sean, et al. *Needle Acupuncture for Posttraumatic Stress Disorder (PTSD)*. PDF ed., RAND, 2017. Research Reports.

25. Nielsen, Arya. "The Science of Acupuncture Safety: Risks, Harms, and Ancient

Goodness." *Pacific College of Oriental Medicine*, Pacific College of Oriental Medicine, 7 Jan. 2019, www.pacificcollege.edu/news/blog/2015/04/27/science-acupuncture-safety-risks-harms-ancient-goodness.

26. "Acupressure for Beginners." *Explore Integrative Medicine*, UCLA Center for East-West Medicine, exploreim.ucla.edu/self-care/acupressure-and-common-acupressure-points/.

27. Hseih, Lisa Li-Chen, et al. "A Randomized Controlled Clinical Trial for Low Back Pain Treated by Acupressure and Physical Therapy." *Preventive Medicine*, vol. 39, no. 1, Aug. 2004, doi:10.1016/j.ypmed.2004.01.036. Abstract.

28. Arai, Young-Chang P et al. "The Influence of Acupressure at Extra 1 Acupuncture Point on the Spectral Entropy of the EEG and the LF/HF Ratio of Heart Rate Variability." *Evidence-based complementary and alternative medicine : eCAM* vol. 2011 (2011): 503698. doi:10.1093/ecam/nen061.

29. Debenedittis, Gluseppe, et al. "Autonomic Changes during Hypnosis: A Heart Rate

Variability Power Spectrum Analysis as a Marker of Sympatho-Vagal Balance." *International Journal of Clinical and Experimental Hypnosis*, vol. 42, no. 2, May 1994, doi:10.1080/00207149408409347. Abstract.

30. Seymour, Tom. "Everything You Need to Know About the Vagus Nerve." *Medical News Today*, MediLexicon International, 28 June 2017, www.medicalnewstoday.com/articles/318128.php.

31. Lin, Wei-Chun, et al. "The Anti-Inflammatory Actions of Auricular Point Acupressure for Chronic Low Back Pain." *Evidence-Based Complementary and Alternative Medicine*, 2015, doi:10.1155/2015/103570.

32. Chrislip, Mark. "Moxibustion." *Science-Based Medicine*, Science-Based Medicine, 18 Apr. 2014, sciencebasedmedicine.org/moxibustion/.

33. Nowakowski, Rachel. "The Healing Power of Moxa." *Daoist Traditions College*, Daoist Traditions College, 5 Oct. 2016, daoisttraditions.edu/healing-power-moxa/.

34. Hafner, Christopher. "Moxibustion." *Taking Charge of Your Health & Wellbeing*, University of Minnesota, www.takingcharge.csh.umn.edu/explore-healing-practices/moxibustion.

35. Song, Xiao-jing, et al. "Analysis of the Spectral Characteristics of Pure Moxa Stick Burning by Hyperspectral Imaging and Fourier Transform Infrared Spectroscopy." *Evidence-based Complementary and Alternative Medicine*, vol. 2016, no. 2, Jan. 2016, doi:10.1155/2016/1057878.

36. Ju, Yan-li, et al. "Forty Cases of Insomnia Treated by Suspended Moxibustion at Baihui (GV 20)." *Journal of Traditional Chinese Medicine*, vol. 29, no. 2, June 2009, doi:10.1016/S0254-6272(09)60040-6.

37. Matsumoto-Miyazaki, Jun, et al. "Traditional Thermal Therapy with Indirect Moxibustion Decreases Renal Arterial Resistive Index in Patients with Chronic Kidney Disease." *The Journal of Alternative and Complementary Medicine*, vol. 22, no. 4, Apr. 2016, doi:10.1089/acm.2015.0276. Abstract.

38. Xu, Ji, et al. "Safety of Moxibustion: A Systematic Review of Case Reports." *Evidence-*

Based Complementary and Alternative Medicine, vol. 2014, May 2014, doi:10.1155/2014/783704.

39. Huizen, Jennifer. "6 Uses of Tiger Balm." *Medical News Today*, MediLexicon International, 22 Nov. 2018, www.medicalnewstoday.com/articles/323771. php.

40. Kotaka, Tomohiko, et al. "Camphor Induces Cold and Warm Sensations with Increases in Skin and Muscle Blood Flow in Human." *Biological and Pharmaceutical Bulletin*, vol. 37, no. 12, Dec. 2014, doi:10.1248/ bpb.b14-00442.

41. Van De Walle, Gavin. "5 Ways to Increase Nitric Oxide Naturally." *Healthline*, Healthline Media, 26 Apr. 2018, www.healthline.com/nutrition/how-to-increase-nitric-oxide.

42. Millqvist, Eva, et al. "Inhalation of Menthol Reduces Capsaicin Cough Sensitivity and Influences Inspiratory Flows in Chronic Cough." *Respiratory Medicine*, vol. 107, no. 3, Mar. 2013, doi:10.1016/j.rmed.2012.11.017.

43. Higashi, Yoshinobu, et al. "Efficacy and Safety Profile of a Topical Methyl Salicylate and Menthol Patch in Adult Patients with

Mild to Moderate Muscle Strain: A Randomized, Double-Blind, Parallel-Group, Placebo-Controlled, Multicenter Study." *Clinical Therapeutics*, vol. 32, no. 1, Jan. 2010, doi:10.1016/j.clinthera.2010.01.016.

44. "Sports Cream Warnings Urged After Teen's Death." *NBC News*, NBC Universal News Group, 13 June 2007, www.nbcnews.com/id/19208195/ns/health-fitness/t/sports-cream-warnings-urged-after-teens-death/#.XTpPd5NKiqC.

45. Qian, Zhang. "TCM Calls for Feet Soaks." *Shanghai Daily*, Shanghai Daily, 21 Jan. 2016, archive.shine.cn/feature/ideal/TCM-calls-for-feet-soaks/shdaily.shtml.

46. Yun, Zhou Xuan. "How Chinese Foot Baths Can Improve Your Health." *Daoist Gate*, 13 Nov. 2016, daoistgate.com/how-chinese-foot-baths-can-improve-your-health/.

47. Anthony, Kiara. "Epsom Salt Foot Soak." Edited by Debra Rose William, *Healthline*, Healthline Media, 29 Apr. 2019, www.healthline.com/health/epsom-salt-foot-soak.

48. Werner, T., et al. "Transdermal Magnesium - 'Myth or Reality'?" *Journal of the Australian Traditional-Medicine Society*, vol. 23, no. 4, Summer 2017, search.informit.com.au/documentSummary;d n=640780639604960;res=IELHEA.

49. "Studies Show Magnesium Reduces Chronic Inflammation, the Cause of Most Chronic Disease." *PR Newswire*, PR Newswire, 29 Oct. 2013, www.prnewswire.com/news-releases/studies-show-magnesium-reduces-chronic-inflammation-the-cause-of-most-chronic-disease-229683651.html.

50. "Warm Water Works Wonders on Pain." *Arthritis Foundation*, Arthritis Foundation, www.arthritis.org/living-with-arthritis/pain-management/tips/warm-water-therapy.php.

51. Leonard, Jayne. "Can You Take Too Much Magnesium?" *Medical News Today*, MediLexicon International, 16 Oct. 2018, www.medicalnewstoday.com/articles/323349.php.

52. "Leg Edema." *Drugs*, www.drugs.com/cg/leg-edema-aftercare-instructions.html.

53. Ingraham, Paul. "Does Epsom Salt Work?" *Pain Science*, Pain Science, 2006, www.painscience.com/articles/epsom-salts.php.

54. Salari, Mohammad Hossein, et al. "Antibacterial Effects of Eucalyptus GlobulusLeaf Extract on Pathogenic Bacteria Isolated from Specimens of Patients with Respiratory Tract Disorders." *Clinical Microbiology and Infection*, vol. 12, no. 2, Feb. 2006, doi:10.1111/j.1469-0691.2005.01284.x. Abstract.

55. Serafino, Annalucia et al. "Stimulatory effect of Eucalyptus essential oil on innate cell-mediated immune response." *BMC immunology* vol. 9 17. 18 Apr. 2008, doi:10.1186/1471-2172-9-17.

56. Bachir, Raho G, and M Benali. "Antibacterial activity of the essential oils from the leaves of Eucalyptus globulus against Escherichia coli and Staphylococcus aureus." *Asian Pacific journal of tropical biomedicine* vol. 2,9 (2012): 739-42. doi:10.1016/S2221-1691(12)60220-2.

57. Jun, Yang Suk, et al. "Effect of Eucalyptus Oil Inhalation on Pain and Inflammatory Responses after Total Knee Replacement: A

Randomized Clinical Trial." *Evidence-Based Complementary and Alternative Medicine*, vol. 2013, 18 June 2013, doi:10.1155/2013/502727.

58. Nordqvist, Joseph. "The Health Benefits of Eucalyptus." *Medical News Today*, MediLexicon International, 5 Jan. 2018, www.medicalnewstoday.com/articles/266580.php.

59. "Essential Oils: Poisonous When Misused." *Poison Control*, National Capital Poison Center, www.poison.org/articles/2014-jun/essential-oils.

60. "Lemongrass." *Memorial Sloan Kettering Cancer Center*, Memorial Sloan Kettering Cancer Center, www.mskcc.org/cancer-care/integrative-medicine/herbs/lemongrass#msk_consumer.

61. Ekpenyong, Christopher E., et al. "Bioactive Natural Constituents from Lemongrass Tea and Erythropoiesis Boosting Effects: Potential Use in Prevention and Treatment of Anemia." *Journal of Medicinal Food*, vol. 18, no. 1, 6 Jan. 2015, doi:10.1089/jmf.2013.0184.

62. Ridzuan, P.M., et al. "Antibacterial and Antifungal Properties of persicaria odorata Leaf Against Pathogenic Bacteria and Fungi." *The Open Conference Proceedings Journal*, vol. 2013, no. 4, 2013, pdfs.semanticscholar.org/7726/841f52fa939d 149568a5dc7a5134c55e299b.pdf.

63. Ware, Megan. "Ginger: Health Benefits and Dietary Tips." *Medical News Today*, MediLexicon International, 11 Sept. 2017, www.medicalnewstoday.com/articles/265990. php.

64. Olsen, Natalie. "Is Drinking Ginger Water Good for Health?" *Medical News Today*, MediLexicon International, 25 June 2018, www.medicalnewstoday.com/articles/322257. php.